THE HEALING POWER OF CAYENNE PEPPER

complete handbook of cayenne home remedies

Patrick Quillin, PhD,RD,CNS

The Leader Co., Inc.
North Canton, OH

Other books by Patrick Quillin, PhD,RD,CNS
available at your local bookstore or health food store.
-BEATING CANCER WITH NUTRITION, Nutrition Times Press,
Tulsa, 1998
-IMMUNOPOWER, Nutrition Times Press, Tulsa, 1998
-KITCHEN HEALTH TIPS, 56 minute videotape, Nutrition Times,
1997
-HONEY, GARLIC & VINEGAR, Home Remedies, Leader Co., N.
Canton, OH, 1996
-HEALTH TIPS, Nutrition Times Press, Tulsa, 1996
-ADJUVANT NUTRITION IN CANCER TREATMENT, Cancer
Treatment Research Foundation, Arlington Heights, IL, 1994
-AMISH FOLK MEDICINE, Leader Co., N.Canton, OH, 1993
-SAFE EATING, M.Evans, NY, 1990
-LA COSTA BOOK OF NUTRITION, Pharos Books, New York,
1988
-HEALING NUTRIENTS, Contemporary Books, Chicago, 1987, in
paperback by Random House, NY, 1988; also published in paperback in
Europe and Australia through Penguin Press, London
-THE LA COSTA PRESCRIPTION FOR LONGER LIFE, Ballantine
Books, NY, 1985

Printed in the United States of America

The Leader Co., Inc.
931 N. Main #101
N. Canton, OH   44720
800-899-6117, 330-494-6988; fax -6989

CONTENTS

Heart disease
Heart arrhythmia
Heat exhaustion
Herbal augmentor
High blood pressure
High cholesterol
Libido
Malnutrition
Mouth sores
Nausea
Obesity
Osteoarthritis
Pain
Pesticide
Pleurisy
Psoriasis
Shingles
Sinusitis
Skin problems
Sore throat
Stress reducer
Stroke
Thyroid problems
Toothache Toxin protection
Ulcers
Urinary tract
Warming effect Worms